CW00542036

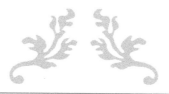

BREVILLE AIR FRYER COOKBOOK FOR BEGINNERS

40 Beginner Recipes To Make Your Meals Light, Healthy And Tasty With The Air Fryer

Carol Evans

this book has been derived from various sources. Please consult a licensed professional before attempting any techniques outlined in this book.

By reading this document, the reader agrees that under no circumstances is the author responsible for any losses, direct or indirect, which are incurred as a result of the use of information contained within this document, including, but not limited to, errors, omissions, or inaccuracies.

Table of Contents

INTRODUCTION 9

BREAKFAST RECIPES 21

   Easy Egg Casserole 22

   Flavor Packed Breakfast Casserole 24

   Vegetable Sausage Egg Bake 26

   Ham Egg Brunch Bake 28

LUNCH RECIPES 31

   Sweet And Sticky Turkey Wings 31

DINNER RECIPES 33

   Sour And Spicy Spareribs 34

   Tender Pork Shoulder With Hot Peppers 36

POULTRY RECIPES 39

   Buffalo Chicken Wings 39

   Zingy & Nutty Chicken Wings 40

   Honey And Wine Chicken Breasts 42

PORK, BEEF & LAMB RECIPES 43

   Chinese Style Pork Chops 44

   Cinco De Mayo Pork Taquitos 46

   Tangy Smoked Pork Chops With Raspberry Sauce 48

   Air fryer toast oven bacon 50

SEAFOOD 51

   Air Fryer Salmon Patties 52

   Fried Calamari 53

   Panko-Crusted Tilapia 54

   Salmon Croquettes 55

VEGETABLES 57

    Mushroom, Onion And Feta Frittata 58

SOUPS AND STEWS 59

    Surprising Sweet Potato Stew 59

SNACKS 61

    Eggplant Milanese 62

BREADS RECIPES 65

    Sunflower Seed Bread 66

    Date Bread 68

    Date & Walnut Bread 70

    Brown Sugar Banana Bread 73

DEHYDRATED RECIPES 75

    Cinnamon Apples Slices 75

    Smoky Eggplant Bacon 76

VEGETARIAN 77

    Beet, Tomato And Goat Cheese Mix 78

    Broccoli Salad 79

    Brussels Sprouts And Tomatoes Mix 80

    Brussels Sprouts And Butter Sauce 81

    Cheesy Brussels Sprouts 82

SNACKS & APPETIZERS 83

    French Fries 83

    Air Fried Pickle 84

    Beef Taquitos 86

    Cheese Sandwich 87

    Perfect Cinnamon Toast 88

DESSERTS... 89

    Vanilla Peanut Butter Cake 90

    Moist Chocolate Brownies.. 92

    Yummy Scalloped Pineapple.. 94

    Vanilla Lemon Cupcakes.. 95

INTRODUCTION

An air fryer is a great kitchen product that saves money and energy. By using a tablespoon of oil and ten minutes it can make the tastiest French fries in the world and help you lose the fatty muffin bottom, too. The product has a flexible mini-oven and there's no risk of splattering oil on your countertops! You'll have crispy breaded items without the grease of a traditional deep fryer. The appliance's splash-guard tray can be removed, and the non-slip feet allow it to sit securely on the counter while cooking.

The highest-rated air fryers on the market can be used to make crispy French fries, chicken tenders, and yummy little steaks. The stainless-steel appliance hooks up to a variety of dishes. The best air fryer has a digital timer and temperature controls. You can also get an air fryer that has a turntable, timer, and a start/stop/ pause control.

Air fryers do not require a lot of oil most recipes call for only a couple tablespoons of oil. If you're using frozen chicken wings, they need more oil to them crispy and juicy. An air fryer is easy to use and clean up after. If you've been trying to get rid of a greasy fryer and a hot, oily kitchen; there is a great solution. Even the best air fryers on the market don't need oil for good taste. You'll get crispy French fries, chicken fingers, and other yummy things. The air fryer is a healthier way of cooking, so you'll look better and feel better.

This guide has 601 affordable and delicious recipes for beginners and advanced users, from breakfast to dinner. Even experienced chefs will adore that the air fryer cooks food to perfection; no need to worry about over oiling, plain food, or food falling apart as it cooks. If you're wanting to lose weight, air fryers can be a smart addition to your kitchen. Cooking helps you to lose weight by creating movement that causes your body to burn calories.

Fast and easy cooking is easy with this single appliance. You can even use it as an oven! The air fryer is safe to use around little ones.

After a few uses of this kitchen gem people will follow you. The air fryer does not require an extra pan or pot to heat up. Steak is a great tasting dish, but not the fastest thing to cook. An air fryer can change that and make that yummy steak for almost instant gratification.

In the past when people had a big family, they needed to cook a lot of food. These days, people have families, but they do not cook as much. The air fryer makes it simple to cook a batch of fresh food for the family so they will feel better about eating healthy. The air fryer can save money. Some frying recipes call for up to a gallon of oil. That oil could go a long way! Spending too much money on food hurts the wallet.

What Is The Breville Air Fryer

Breville Air Fryer is nothing but a revolutionary innovation in the process of frying and is a user-friendly product. It is basically a frying machine which can dry, bake or roast food by using hot air and it does not need any oil, whereas it doesn't add any oil to food either. This means that the food you're frying remain free of oil and calories.

How Use A Breville Air Fryer

Before you know use a Breville Air Fryer is that you need to do some preparations before you use it and you need to keep some precautions into account. A simple illustration of how to use a Breville air fryer is that you need to fill in it with the oil and it will be good enough for you to cook something for family members or friends.

Steps to Use a Breville Air Fryer

• The first thing to use a Breville air fryer is to press the power button and then lock the handle whatever texture you are cooking.

• Make sure the basket is locked and the temperature will be heated automatically.

• Make sure to put your food into the basket and use a utensil to turn it over to check all sides are cooked.

• You need to keep the air flow.

• Make sure to empty the basket after it is cooked and put it in the dishwasher.

Users will start to love a Breville air fryer since they are easy to use and to clean. No extra oil is needed to be added since the air fryer has an excellent function of floating the oil around to cook the quality of the food..

here are some of the functions of a breville air fryer:

• Non-stick basket – offers 100% of the protection against wire marks or scratches.

• Electronic touchpad controls – easy to access and operate, with a timer.

• Separate temperature dial – allows you to set different temperatures for your chips, veggies, chicken , fish and etc.

• Power basket – great option for moving foods from one frying compartment to the next.

• Food holder – easy to use and hold.

• Extra functions – includes a ready alert, lockable handle, automatic shut-off, and dishwasher-safe parts.

How To Prepare The Smart Oven For The First Use

After you receive the order of air fryer, the first thing you need to do is to open the box. Make sure that you remove all the packing materials and protective covers. Moreover, remove all the accessories from the box but do not mix them. It is advised not to install the device until you have set it to the packaging provided. The gadget cannot be used for frying until it is fully assembled. Ensure all the parts have been connected properly; you can have F-cups for everything. The air fryer instructions for using an electric air fryer are given below.

1. Take the metal rack out and add it to your F-cup. This F-cup shines brighter than the rest so it is easily distinguished.

2. Take the grill net or tray out of the box and place it in the F-cup you've ironed for the rack.

3. Place the heavy base on the F-cup where you've placed the grill net.

4. Pour in the recommended amount of vegetable oil.

5. Your new oven is now ready for use.

Functions Of The Smart Air Fryer

The air fryer has a number of features that makes it easy to use and fun. The device is programmed in such a way that it starts heating on its own at whatever time you set it too. This may be in the morning as you are getting ready for work, or in the evening while you are ready to get dinner started for your family. The air fryer uses the same amount of time to heat up to 320 degrees as it would normally when using this high heat for the actual cooking of a meal. This means that fuel usage is cut down, saving money in the long run. No more rushing to get the food cooked, this air fryer lets you actually make sure it is ready in the morning, so you have all day to spend at work. The thought of getting that smell of breakfast cooking or dinner as you walk through the door is almost as good as the food itself.

Here are some of the functions of a smart air fryer:

Toast- The air fryer toasts bread, bagels and food a like to the perfect toasty brown.

Air Fry- Pushing a button and the air fryer is programmed to heat up to 320 degrees, cook and then cool down. There is a timer that allows the air fryer to shut off at a pre-set amount of time. This allows you to cook food without having to worry about the time. You can set it and forget it, like you would when using a microwave.

Bagel- Air fryers let you toast, bagel and broil all in one appliance.

Broil- Broil perfectly golden brown with delicious dry heat with the air fryer.

Bake- No more cooking with grease or oil, with the air fryer bake perfectly like a fresh out of the oven batch of goodies.

Roast- The air fryer allows you to cook up perfectly browned roasts that are cooked to perfection without having to open the oven for a peek.

Warm- Warm herbed rolls, pork chops, vegetables, ribs and hot dogs with the air fryer.

Pizza- Cook all the favorite pizza toppings to a yummy golden brown.

Proof- Bake yeast rolls and dough just like the bakeries of old do.

Air Fry- The air fryer gives golden, crispy fried foods with little or no oil. Nothing dipped, breaded, floured or fried? No problem, still easy and the ultimate in fat free cooking.

Reheat- To warm up already cooked foods, there is no need to fire up the oven and make things even hotter. The air fryer can be set for a timer of any length to warm-up already cooked foods.

Cookies- Cookies crisp wonderfully within the heated air of the air fryer.

Slow Cook- As you move around your home using your air fryer, cook soups, sauces, stews and casseroles without having to watch and stir, thanks to the convenient slow cook setting.

Dehydrate- A dehydrator no longer needed. Place fruit, kale and so on into the air fryer and let it do all the work of dehydrating all the food you have.

The air fryer is health conscious cooking with a little added spice, without the added fat that lets you get the same great taste and warm smell as using your regular cookware.

Benefits On Using This Air Fryer

Some of the basic benefits of using this air fryer are:

• Reduced Cooking Time : The air fryer expands the amount of heat so that the food turns out crispy faster and quicker.

• Healthy Cooking: The air fryer uses less oil and is healthier for people. The oils used to cook French fries or other fried favorites disappear in the outer rings and not inside the food.

• Safe to Use: The energy-efficient design is much safer than a conventional fryer. There are no open flames or hot pots of oil.

• Trouble-Free Cleanup: The oil-less air fryers allow snack foods to be prepared without transferring any oil to the kitchen. It is mess-free due to the absence of oil.

• Flavorful Snacks: The air fryer doesn't use oil, so it doesn't add a greasy factor to food. The air fryer can be used to prepare fish, chicken, vegetables, and different kinds of appetizers as well.

• No Oiling Required: Unlike traditional deep-fryers, air fryers don't require oil because they don't need to be immersed in oil. They need just the right amount of oil in between the food items, with the food being put in first.

• Smooth Health: The process of deep-frying in oil is a dangerous health hazard, as it can cause heart problems and other complications for people who consume a lot of this oily food. The air fryer has eliminated this risk.

• Healthier Alternative: The air fryer only requires a small amount of oil to create crispy and golden-brown fried treats. Without oil, fried foods can be healthier options.

• Crispier Food: The air fryer can retain the crispiness factor in the foods it fries, with less oil than grease needs.

• Versatile: An air fryer can create a wide variety of foods such as vegetables, chicken, fish, shrimp, and anything else that can be deep-fried.

• Easily Available: The air fryer only comes in one size, and can be used for deep-frying , baking, and convection heating. The air fryer comes with a variety of accessories and a recipe book of various things that can be prepared in it.

• Easily Cleaned: After a delicious meal is prepared in the air fryer, it can be cleaned very easily. The air fryer has a very easy cleaning process.

• Space Saving: Air fryers are very small and can be stored easily in any space. They take up a very small footprint when compared to deep fryers.

How To Clean And Take Care Of This Air Fryer

Cleaning and maintenance of an air fryer is very easy and simple. But even then, it is recommended to do it every time you use it. It ensures safety and efficiency of the appliance. And you can easily clean it. To clean your air fryer follow these steps:

1. Open the lid, untie the food tray and discard it.

2. Fill the fryer with warm water and put the food tray and base into the water.

3. Stir the water to mix the oil and food.

4. Leave it for 10 minutes.

5. You can see the oil rising in the water. When the oil stops rising.

6. Take the food tray and base out of the water and rinse the food tray with warm water.

7. If you see oil in the base insert the base rotating it 15 degrees or half a turn.

8. Then you should be able to see the hole at the center of the base and use the pump or a pipe cleaner with water to get the remaining oil.

9. After cleaning the oil, put the food tray and base inside the air fryer again.

10. Add warm water again and then wait for 15 minutes inside the air fryer.

11. After 15 minutes, you can take the food tray and base out to dry them.

12. After the food tray and base are dry, use the vacuum cleaner to clean the interior of the air fryer.

13. Then, clean the lid, the base and the food tray with warm water.

Keeping your air fryer clean is very easy. As it is very clean and hygienic. Keeping it clean not only helps increase its life but also makes it work efficiently.

BREAKFAST RECIPES

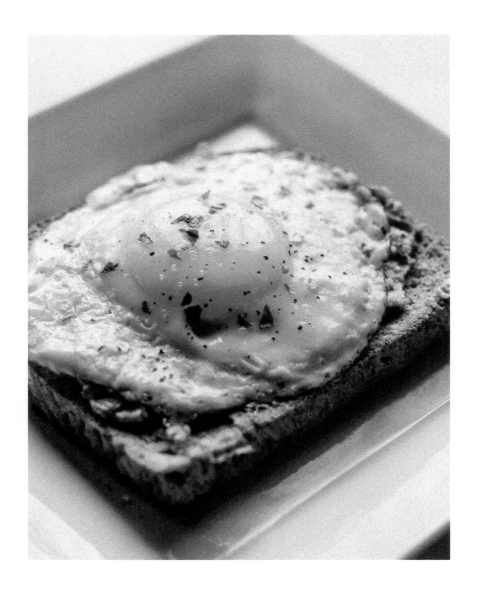

Easy Egg Casserole

Preparation time: 10 minutes

Cooking time: 55 minutes

Servings: 8

Ingredients:

- 8 eggs
- 1/2 tsp garlic powder
- 2 cups cheddar cheese, shredded
- 1 cup milk
- 24 oz frozen hash browns, thawed
- 1/2 onion, diced
- 1 red pepper, diced
- 4 bacon slices, diced
- 1/2 lb turkey breakfast sausage
- Pepper
- Salt

Directions:

1. Spray a 9*13-inch baking dish with cooking spray and set aside.
2. Insert wire rack in rack position 6. Select bake, set temperature 350 f, timer for 50 minutes. Press start to preheat the oven.

3. Cook breakfast sausage in a pan over medium heat until cooked through. Drain well and set aside.

4. Cook bacon in the same pan. Drain well and set aside.

5. In a mixing bowl, whisk eggs with milk, garlic powder, pepper, and salt. Add 1 cup cheese, hash browns, onion, red pepper, bacon, and sausage and stir well.

6. Pour the entire egg mixture into the baking dish. Sprinkle remaining cheese on top.

7. Cover dish with foil and bake for 50 minutes. Remove foil and bake for 5 minutes more.

8. Serve and enjoy.

Nutrition: Calories 479 Fat 29.1 g Carbohydrates 34.1 g Sugar 4.2 g Protein 20.2 g Cholesterol 207 mg

Flavor Packed Breakfast Casserole

Preparation time: 10 minutes

Cooking time: 40 minutes

Servings: 8

Ingredients:

- 12 eggs
- 1/2 cup cheddar cheese, shredded
- 1 tsp garlic powder
- 1 cup milk
- 1/4 cup onion, diced
- 2 bell pepper, cubed
- 4 small potatoes, cubed
- 2 cups sausage, cooked and diced
- Pepper
- Salt

Directions:

1. Spray a 9*13-inch baking dish with cooking spray and set aside.
2. Insert wire rack in rack position 6. Select bake, set temperature 350 f, timer for 40 minutes. Press start to preheat the oven.

3. In a large bowl, whisk eggs with milk, garlic powder, pepper, and salt.

4. Add sausage, bell peppers, and potatoes into the baking dish. Pour egg mixture over sausage mixture. Sprinkle with cheese and onion.

5. Bake casserole for 40 minutes.

6. Slice and serve.

Nutrition: Calories 232 Fat 11.6 g Carbohydrates 18.3 g Sugar 4.6 g Protein 14.2 g Cholesterol 261 mg

Vegetable Sausage Egg Bake

Preparation time: 10 minutes

Cooking time: 35 minutes

Servings: 4

Ingredients:

- 10 eggs
- 1 cup spinach, diced
- 1 cup onion, diced
- 1 cup pepper, diced
- 1 lb sausage, cut into 1/2-inch pieces
- 1 tsp garlic powder
- 1/2 cup almond milk
- Pepper
- Salt

Directions:

1. Spray an 8*8-inch baking dish with cooking spray and set aside.
2. Insert wire rack in rack position 6. Select bake, set temperature 390 f, timer for 35 minutes. Press start to preheat the oven.
3. In a bowl, whisk eggs with milk and spices. Add vegetables and sausage and stir to combine.

4. Pour egg mixture into the prepared baking dish. Bake for 35 minutes.

5. Slice and serve.

Nutrition: Calories 653 Fat 50.6 g Carbohydrates 12.6 g Sugar 3.3 g Protein 38.3 g Cholesterol 504 mg

Ham Egg Brunch Bake

Preparation time: 10 minutes

Cooking time: 60 minutes

Servings: 6

Ingredients:

- 4 eggs
- 20 oz hash browns
- 1 onion, chopped
- 2 cups ham, chopped
- 3 cups cheddar cheese, shredded
- 1 cup sour cream
- 1 cup milk
- Pepper
- Salt

Directions:

1. Spray a 9*13-inch baking dish with cooking spray and set aside.
2. Insert wire rack in rack position 6. Select bake, set temperature 375 f, timer for 35 minutes. Press start to preheat the oven.
3. In a large mixing bowl, whisk eggs with sour cream, milk, pepper, and salt. Add 2 cups cheese and stir well.
4. Cook onion and ham in a medium pan until onion is softened.

28

5. Add hash brown to the pan and cook for 5 minutes.

6. Add onion ham mixture into the egg mixture and mix well.

7. Pour egg mixture into the prepared baking dish. Cover dish with foil and bake for 35 minutes.

8. Remove foil and bake for 25 minutes more.

9. Slice and serve.

Nutrition: Calories 703 Fat 46.2 g Carbohydrates 41.2 g Sugar 4.6 g Protein 30.8 g Cholesterol 214 mg

LUNCH RECIPES

Sweet And Sticky Turkey Wings

Preparation time: 10 Minutes

Cooking time :20 Minutes

 Servings: 2

Ingredients:

- 1 lbs turkey wings
- ½ teaspoon sea salt
- ¼ cup coconut amino
- ¼ teaspoon ginger minced
- 1teaspoon onion, chopped
- ¼ teaspoon garlic minced
- ¼ teaspoon chili flakes

Directions:

1. Preheat your air fryer to 360 degrees fahrenheit.
2. Sprinkle the wings liberally with fine sea salt
3. Air fry on 360 degrees fahrenheit for 1 hour, turning every 15 minutes or until internal temperature has reached a temperature of 165 degrees fahrenheit.
4. Heat a medium to large skillet over medium heat, and add the coconut amino.

5. Add the minced ginger , minced garlic ,chopped onion , and red pepper flakes (if desired). Once the sauce is simmering, start stirring. Keep stirring at regular intervals and adjust the heat as needed to keep cooking soft.

6. Once the sauce has thickened slightly. Place the wings in a large heatproof bowl, and pour the sauce over them. Stir to coat and serve with sauce!

Nutrition: Calories 123, total fat 5g, total carbohydrate 6.4g, protein 11.5g

DINNER RECIPES

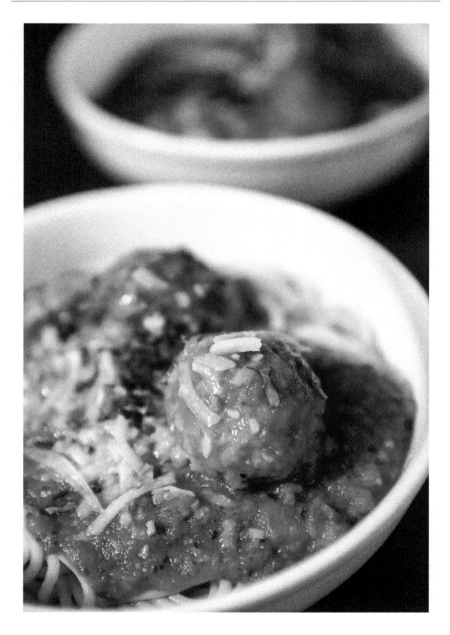

Sour And Spicy Spareribs

Preparation time: 15 minutes

Cooking time: 35 minutes

Servings: 10

Ingredients:

- 5 lbs. Spare spareribs
- Salt and pepper to taste
- 2 tbsp. Of tallow
- 1/2 cup coconut amines (from coconut sap)
- 1/2 cup vinegar
- 2 tbsp. Worcestershire sauce, to taste
- 1 tsp. Chili powder
- 1 tsp. Garlic powder
- 1 tsp. Celery seeds

Directions:

1. Cut the rack of ribs into equal portions.
2. Season salt and ground pepper your spareribs from all sides.
3. Add tallow in your instant pot and place spareribs.
4. In a bowl, combine all remaining ingredients: and pour over spareribs.
5. Lock lid into place and set on the manual setting on high heat for 35 minutes.

6. When the timer beeps, press "cancel" and carefully flip the natural release for 20 minutes.

7. Open the lid and transfer ribs on a serving platter.

8. Serve hot.

Nutrition: Calories: 598 kcal/cal Carbohydrates: 2 g Proteins: 36 g Fat: 54 g Fiber: 0.2 g

Tender Pork Shoulder With Hot Peppers

Preparation time: 10 minutes

Cooking time: 30 minutes

Servings: 8

Ingredients:

- 3 lbs. Pork shoulder boneless
- Salt and ground black pepper to taste
- 3 tbsp. Of olive oil
- 1 large onion, chopped
- 2 cloves garlic minced
- 2 - 3 chili peppers, chopped
- 1 tsp. Ground coriander
- 1 tsp. Ground cumin
- 1 ½ cups of bone broth (preferably homemade)
- 1/2 cup water

Directions:

1. Season salt and pepper the pork meat.
2. Turn on the instant pot and press sauté button. When the word "hot" appears on the display, add the oil and sauté the onions and garlic about 5 minutes.
3. Add pork and sear for 1 - 2 minutes from all sides; turn off the sauté button.

4. Add all remaining ingredients into instant pot.

5. Lock lid into place and set on the meat/stew setting on high heat for 30 minutes.

6. When the timer beeps, press "cancel" and carefully flip the natural release button for 15 minutes. Serve hot.

Nutrition: Calories: 389 kcal/cal Carbohydrates: 2.5 g Proteins: 36 g Fat: 27 g Fiber: 0.5 g

POULTRY RECIPES

Buffalo Chicken Wings

Preparation time: 5 minutes

Cooking time: 30 minutes

Servings: 8

Ingredients:

- 1 tsp. Salt
- 1-2 tbsp. Brown sugar
- 1 tbsp. Worcestershire sauce
- ½ c. Vegan butter
- ½ c. Cayenne pepper sauce
- 4 pounds chicken wings

Directions:

1. Whisk salt, brown sugar, worcestershire sauce, butter, and hot sauce together and set to the side.
2. Dry wings and add to air fryer basket.
3. Set temperature to 380°f, and set time to 25 minutes. Cook tossing halfway through.
4. When timer sounds, shake wings and bump up the temperature to 400 degrees and cook another 5 minutes.
5. Take out wings and place into a big bowl. Add sauce and toss well.
6. Serve alongside celery sticks.

Nutrition: calories: 402; fat: 16g; protein:17g; sugar:4g

Zingy & Nutty Chicken Wings

Preparation time: 5 minutes

Cooking time: 18 minutes

Servings: 4

Ingredients:

- 1 tablespoon fish sauce

- 1 tablespoon fresh lemon juice

- 1 teaspoon sugar

- 12 chicken middle wings, cut into half

- 2 fresh lemongrass stalks, chopped finely

- ¼ cup unsalted cashews, crushed

Directions:

1. In a bowl, mix together fish sauce, lime juice and sugar.

2. Add wings ad coat with mixture generously. Refrigerate to marinate for about 1-2 hours.

3. Preheat the cuisinart air fryer oven to 355 degrees f.

4. In the cuisinart air fryer oven pan, place lemongrass stalks. Cook for about 2-3 minutes. Remove the cashew mixture from air fryer and transfer into a bowl. Now, set the cuisinart air fryer oven to 390 degrees f.

5. Place the chicken wings in air fryer pan. Cook for about 13-15 minutes further.
6. Transfer the wings into serving plates. Sprinkle with cashew mixture and serve.

Nutrition: Calories: 356; Fat: 26g; Protein:23g; Sugar:2g

Honey And Wine Chicken Breasts

Preparation time: 5 minutes

Cooking time: 15 minutes

Servings: 4

Ingredients:

- 2 chicken breasts, rinsed and halved
- 1 tablespoon melted butter
- 1/2 teaspoon freshly ground pepper, or to taste
- 3/4 teaspoon sea salt, or to taste
- 1 teaspoon paprika
- 1 teaspoon dried rosemary
- 2 tablespoons dry white wine
- 1 tablespoon honey

Directions:

1. Firstly, pat the chicken breasts dry. Lightly coat them with the melted butter.
2. Then, add the remaining ingredients.
3. Transfer them to the air fryer basket; bake about 15 minutes at 330 degrees f. Serve warm and enjoy!

Nutrition: calories: 189; fat: 14g; protein:11g; sugar:1g

PORK, BEEF & LAMB RECIPES

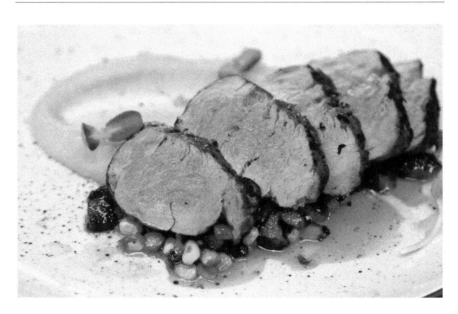

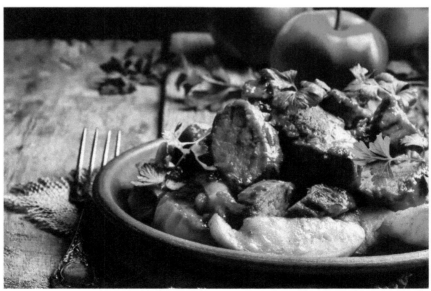

Chinese Style Pork Chops

Preparation time: 15 minutes

Cooking time: 20 minutes

Servings: 4

Ingredients:

- 450g pork chops
- ¾ cup corn/potato starch
- 1 egg white
- ¼ tsp. Freshly ground black pepper
- ½ tsp. Kosher salt
- For the stir fry:
- 2 green onions, sliced
- 2 jalapeno peppers, seeds removed and sliced
- 2 tbsp. Peanut oil
- ¼ tsp. Freshly ground pepper and kosher salt to taste

Directions:

1. Brush or spray the basket of your air fryer toast oven with oil.
2. Next, whisk the egg, black pepper and salt until it gets frothy. Cut up the pork chops and use a clean kitchen towel to pat the meat dry.
3. Toss the cutlets in the frothy egg mixture until evenly coated. Cover and marinate for 30 minutes.

4. Place the pork chops in a separate bowl and pour in the corn/ potato starch ensuring each culet is thoroughly dredged. Shake off the excess corn/ potato starch and arrange the pork chops on the prepared basket.

5. Set the air fryer toast oven at 360 degrees f and cook for 9 minutes, shaking the basket after every 2-3 minutes and spraying or brushing the cutlets with more oil if needed.

6. Increase the temperature to 400 degrees f and cook for 6 more minutes or until the chops are crisp and done to desire.

7. Heat a wok or pan over high heat until extremely hot. Add all the stir fry ingredients: and sauté for a minute.

8. Add your cooked pork chops and toss with the stir fry.

9. Cook for another minute ensuring the pork chops are evenly coated with the stir fry ingredients. Enjoy!

Nutrition: calories: 398 kcal, carbs: 16.1 g, fat: 17.5 g, protein: 21.1 g.

Cinco De Mayo Pork Taquitos

Preparation time: 20 minutes

Cooking time: 15 minutes

Servings: 5

Ingredients:

- 400g cooked and shredded pork tenderloin
- 10 flour tortillas2 ½ cups mozzarella, shredded
- 1 lemon, juiced
- Sour cream
- Salsa
- Cooking spray

Directions:

1. Set your air fryer toast oven to 380 degrees f.
2. Squeeze the lemon juice over the shredded pork and mix well to combine.
3. Divide the tortillas into two and microwave, i batch at a time, covered with a slightly damp paper towel, so they don't become hard, for 15 seconds.
4. Divide the pork and cheese among the 10 tortillas.
5. Gently but tightly roll up all the tortillas.
6. Line your air fryer toast oven's pan with kitchen foil and arrange the tortillas on the pan.

7. Spray the tortillas with the cooking spray and cook for about 10 minutes, turning them over halfway through cook time.

8. Serve hot and enjoy!

Nutrition: calories: 276 kcal, carbs: 12.5 g, fat: 33.9 g, protein: 22.6 g.

Tangy Smoked Pork Chops With Raspberry Sauce

Preparation time: 15 minutes

Cooking time: 25 minutes

Servings: 4

Ingredients:

- 4 medium-sized smoked pork chops
- 1 cup panko bread crumbs
- 2 eggs
- ¼ cup all-purpose flour
- ¼ cup milk
- 1 cup pecans, finely chopped
- 1/3 cup aged balsamic vinegar
- 2 tbsp. Raspberry jam, seedless
- 1 tbsp. Orange juice concentrate
- 2 tbsp. Brown sugar

Directions:

1. Set your air fryer toast oven to 400 degrees f and lightly spray/ brush the basket of your air fryer toast oven with oil.
2. Use a fork to combine the milk and eggs.
3. In a separate bowl, mix the panko bread crumbs with the finely chopped pecan and put the flour in a different bowl.

4. Coat, one pork chop at a time, with flour, shaking any excess off.

5. Next, dunk in the milk mixture and gently coat all sides with the crumb mixture. Pat gently to help the crumbs adhere to the pork chops.

6. Arrange the pork chops in one layer in the prepared basket, spray lightly with cooking oil and cook for about 15 minutes, flipping the chops halfway through cook time.

7. As the chops are cooking, combine all the remaining ingredients in a pan over low-medium heat. Bring to a boil then simmer for 5-8 minutes until it thickens.

8. Take out the chops and serve hot with the raspberry sauce.

9. Enjoy!

Nutrition: calories: 307 kcal, carbs: 31.2 g, fat: 9.1 g, protein: 25.8 g.

Air fryer toast oven bacon

Preparation time: 5 minutes

Cooking time: 15 minutes

Servings: 6

Ingredients:

- 1/2 package (16 ounce) bacon

Directions:

1. Preheat your air fryer toast oven to 390□ f.
2. Arrange the bacon in a single layer in the fryer basket and cook for 8 minutes.
3. Flip over the bacon and cook for 7 minutes more or until crisp.
4. Transfer to a paper lined plate to drain excess grease.
5. Enjoy warm!

Nutrition: calories: 173 kcal, carbs: 0.2 g, fat: 17 g, protein: 4.4 g.

SEAFOOD

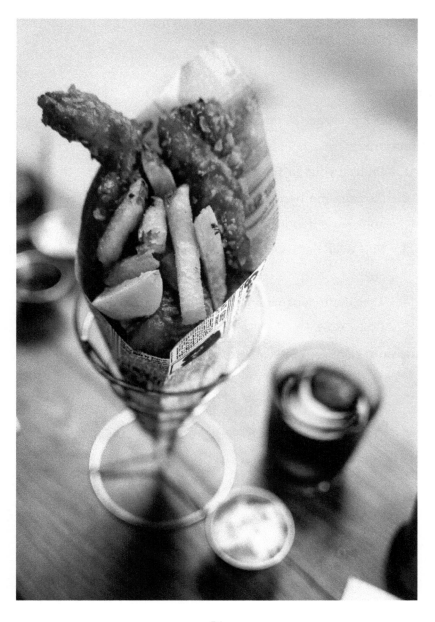

Air Fryer Salmon Patties

Preparation time: 15 minutes

Cooking time: 7 minutes

Servings: 4

Ingredients:

- 1 tbsp. Olive oil
- 1 tbsp. Ghee
- ¼ tsp. Salt
- 1/8 tsp. Pepper
- 1 egg
- 1 c. Almond flour
- 1 cans wild alaskan pink salmon

Directions:

1. Drain can of salmon into a bowl and keeps liquid. Discard skin and bones.
2. Add salt, pepper, and egg to salmon, mixing well with hands to incorporate. Make patties.
3. Dredge in flour and remaining egg. If it seems dry, spoon reserved salmon liquid from the can onto patties.
4. Add patties to air fryer. Cook 7 minutes at 378 degrees till golden, making sure to flip once during cooking process.

Nutrition: calories: 437 carbs: 55 fat 12g protein 24g sugar 2g

Fried Calamari

Preparation time: 15 minutes

Cooking time: 15 minutes

Servings: 8

Ingredients:

- ½ tsp. Salt
- ½ tsp. Old bay seasoning
- 1/3 cup plain cornmeal
- ½ cup semolina flour
- ½ cup almond flour
- 5-6 cup olive oil
- 1 ½ pounds baby squid

Directions:

1. Rinse squid in cold water and slice tentacles, keeping just ¼-inch of the hood in one piece.

2. Combine 1-2 pinches of pepper, salt, old bay seasoning, cornmeal, and both flours together. Dredge squid pieces into flour mixture and place into air fryer. Spray liberally with olive oil.

3. Cook 15 minutes at 345 degrees till coating turns a golden brown.

Nutrition: calories: 211 fat 6g protein 21g sugar 1g

Panko-Crusted Tilapia

Preparation time: 5 minutes

Cooking time: 11 minutes

Servings: 3

Ingredients:

- 2 tsp. Italian seasoning
- 2 tsp. Lemon pepper
- 1/3 cup panko breadcrumbs
- 1/3 cup egg whites
- 1/3 cup almond flour
- 3 tilapia fillets
- Olive oil

Directions:

1. Place panko, egg whites, and flour into separate bowls. Mix lemon pepper and italian seasoning in with breadcrumbs. Pat tilapia fillets dry. Dredge in flour, then egg, then breadcrumb mixture. Add to air fryer basket and spray lightly with olive oil. Cook 10-11 minutes at 400 degrees, making sure to flip halfway through cooking.

Nutrition: calories: 256 fat 9g protein 39g sugar 5g

Salmon Croquettes

Preparation time: 15 minutes

Cooking time: 10 minutes

Servings: 8

Ingredients:

- Panko breadcrumbs
- Almond flour
- 2 egg whites
- 2 tbsp. Chopped chives
- 2 tbsp. Minced garlic cloves
- ½ c. Chopped onion
- 2/3 c. Grated carrots
- 1 pound chopped salmon fillet

Directions:

1. Mix together all ingredients: minus breadcrumbs, flour, and egg whites.
2. Shape mixture into balls. Then coat them in flour, then egg, and then breadcrumbs. Drizzle with olive oil.
3. Add coated salmon balls to air fryer and cook 6 minutes at 350 degrees. Shake and cook an additional 4 minutes until golden in color.

Nutrition: calories: 503 carbs: 61g fat 9g protein 5g sugar 4g

VEGETABLES

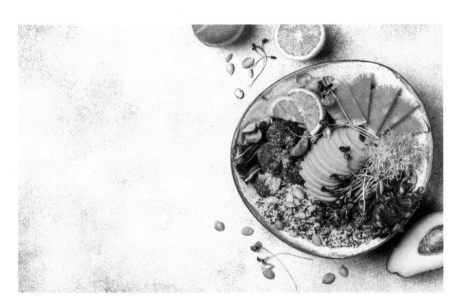

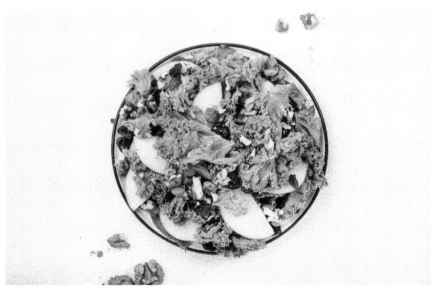

Mushroom, Onion And Feta Frittata

Preparation time: 5 minutes

Cooking time: 30 minutes

Servings: 4

Ingredients:

- 4 cups button mushrooms
- 1 red onion
- 2 tablespoons olive oil
- 6 tablespoons feta cheese, crumbled
- Pinch of salt
- 6 eggs
- Cooking spray

Directions:

1. Peel and slice the red onion into ¼ inch thin slices. Clean the button mushrooms, then cut them into ¼ inch thin slices. Add olive oil to pan and sauté mushrooms over medium heat until tender. Remove from heat and pan so that they can cool. Preheat your air fryer to 330° fahrenheit. Add cracked eggs into a bowl, and whisk them, adding a pinch of salt. Coat an 8-inch heat resistant baking dish with cooking spray. Add the eggs into the baking dish, then onion and mushroom mixture, and then add feta cheese. Place the baking dish into air fryer for 30-minutes and serve warm.

Nutrition: calories: 246 total fat: 12.3g carbohydrates: 9.2g protein: 10.3g

SOUPS AND STEWS

Surprising Sweet Potato Stew

Preparation time: 10-20 minutes

Cooking time: 40 minutes

Servings: 4

Ingredients:

- 1 sweet potato, cubed
- 1 big onion; chopped.
- 1/2 cup red lentils
- 3 garlic cloves; chopped.
- 1 celery stalk; chopped.
- 2 cups veggie stock
- 1/4 cup raisins
- 2 carrots; chopped
- 1 cup green lentils
- 14 oz. Canned tomatoes; chopped.
- Salt and black pepper to the taste
- For the spice blend:
- 1/2 tsp. Cinnamon
- 1/4 tsp. Ginger, grated
- 1 tsp. Cumin
- 1 tsp. Paprika

- 2 tsp. Coriander
- 1 tsp. Turmeric
- A pinch of cloves
- A pinch of chili flakes

Directions:

1. Set your instant pot on sauté mode; add onions and brown them for 2 minutes adding some of the stock from time to time

2. Add garlic, stir and cook for 1 minute

3. Add carrots, raisins, celery, and sweet potatoes, stir and cook for 1 minute.

4. Add red and green lentils, stock, tomatoes, salt, pepper, turmeric, cinnamon, paprika, cumin, coriander, ginger, cloves and chili flakes; then stir well. Seal the instant pot lid and cook at high for 15 minutes.

5. Release the pressure naturally for 15 minutes, then release remaining pressure by turning the valve to 'venting', carefully open the lid; stir stew one more time, add more salt and pepper if needed, ladle into bowls and serve

Nutrition: calories: 230 fat: 5 g protein:1 g

SNACKS

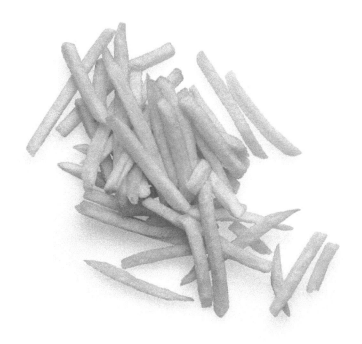

Eggplant Milanese

Preparation time: 5 minutes.

Cooking time: 40 minutes.

Servings: 2

Ingredients:

- 1 medium eggplant
- 1 tbsp of vinegar
- 2 lightly beaten whole eggs
- 1 cup of tea flour
- 1 ½ cup breadcrumbs

Directions:

1. Wash the eggplants and cut into slices of 1 cm maximum thickness, place the slices in a bowl with water and vinegar and let them soak for at least 15 minutes.
2. Preheat the air fryer. Set the time of 5 minutes and the temperature to 200 degrees.
3. Remove water from eggplant slices and place on a roasting pan, sprinkle salt to taste. Pass each slice through the flour, then through the beaten egg and finally in breadcrumbs and squeezing the fingers and hands, so they remain very compact.

4. Place the eggplant slices in the basket of the air fryer and set the timer for 18 minutes and press the power button. Open the time in half to see if the weather needs an adjustment because the eggplants should be crispy on the outside and soft on the inside.

Nutrition: calories: 103 fat: 5.61g carbohydrates: 11.61g protein: 2.4g

BREADS RECIPES

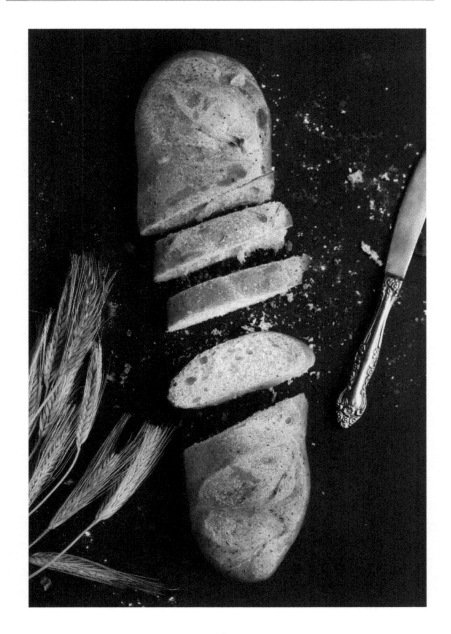

Sunflower Seed Bread

Preparation time: 15 minutes

Cooking time: 18 minutes

Servings: 6

Ingredients:

- 2/3 cup whole-wheat flour
- 2/3 cup plain flour
- 1/3 cup sunflower seeds
- ½ sachet instant yeast
- 1 teaspoon salt
- 2/3-1 cup lukewarm water

Directions:

1. In a bowl, mix together the flours, sunflower seeds, yeast, and salt.
2. Slowly, add in the water, stirring continuously until a soft dough ball forms.
3. Now, move the dough onto a lightly floured surface and knead for about 5 minutes using your hands.
4. Make a ball from the dough and place into a bowl.
5. With a plastic wrap, cover the bowl and place at a warm place for about 30 minutes.
6. Grease a cake pan.
7. Coat the top of dough with water and place into the prepared cake pan.

8. Press "power button" of air fry oven and turn the dial to select the "air crisp" mode.

9. Press the time button and again turn the dial to set the cooking time to 18 minutes.

10. Now push the temp button and rotate the dial to set the temperature at 390 degrees f.

11. Press "start/pause" button to start.

12. When the unit beeps to show that it is preheated, open the lid.

13. Arrange the pan in "air fry basket" and insert in the oven.

14. Place the pan onto a wire rack to cool for about 10 minutes.

15. Carefully, invert the bread onto wire rack to cool completely before slicing.

16. Cut the bread into desired-sized slices and serve.

Nutrition: Calories 132 Total fat 1.7 g Saturated fat 0.1 g Cholesterol 0 mg Sodium 390 mg Total carbs 24.4 g

Fiber 1.6 g Sugar 0.1 g Protein 4.9 g

Date Bread

Preparation time: 15 minutes

Cooking time: 22 minutes

Servings: 10

Ingredients:

- 2½ cup dates, pitted and chopped
- ¼ cup butter
- 1 cup hot water
- 1½ cups flour
- ½ cup brown sugar
- 1 teaspoon baking powder
- 1 teaspoon baking soda
- ½ teaspoon salt
- 1 egg

Directions:

1. In a large bowl, add the dates, butter and top with the hot water.
2. Set aside for about 5 minutes.
3. In another bowl, mix together the flour, brown sugar, baking powder, baking soda, and salt.
4. In the same bowl of dates, mix well the flour mixture, and egg.
5. Grease a baking pan.
6. Place the mixture into the prepared pan.

7. Press "power button" of air fry oven and turn the dial to select the "air crisp" mode.
8. Press the time button and again turn the dial to set the cooking time to 22 minutes.
9. Now push the temp button and rotate the dial to set the temperature at 340 degrees f.
10. Press "start/pause" button to start.
11. When the unit beeps to show that it is preheated, open the lid.
12. Arrange the pan in "air fry basket" and insert in the oven.
13. Place the pan onto a wire rack to cool for about 10 minutes.
14. Carefully, invert the bread onto wire rack to cool completely before slicing.
15. Cut the bread into desired-sized slices and serve.

Nutrition: Calories 269 Total fat 5.4 g Saturated fat 3.1 g Cholesterol 29 mg Sodium 285 mg Total carbs 55.1 g Fiber 4.1 g Sugar 35.3 g Protein 3.6 g

Date & Walnut Bread

Preparation time: 15 minutes

Cooking time: 35 minutes

Servings: 5

Ingredients:

- 1 cup dates, pitted and sliced
- ¾ cup walnuts, chopped
- 1 tablespoon instant coffee powder
- 1 tablespoon hot water
- 1¼ cups plain flour
- ¼ teaspoon salt
- ½ teaspoon baking powder
- ½ teaspoon baking soda
- ½ cup condensed milk
- ½ cup butter, softened
- ½ teaspoon vanilla essence

Directions:

1. In a large bowl, add the dates, butter and top with the hot water.
2. Set aside for about 30 minutes.

3. Drain well and set aside.

4. In a small bowl, add the coffee powder and hot water and mix well.

5. In a large bowl, mix together the flour, baking powder, baking soda and salt.

6. In another large bowl, add the condensed milk and butter and beat until smooth.

7. Add the flour mixture, coffee mixture and vanilla essence and mix until well combined.

8. Fold in dates and ½ cup of walnut.

9. Line a baking pan with a lightly greased parchment paper.

10. Place the mixture into the prepared pan and sprinkle with the remainng walnuts.

11. Press "power button" of air fry oven and turn the dial to select the "air crisp" mode.

12. Press the time button and again turn the dial to set the cooking time to 35 minutes.

13. Now push the temp button and rotate the dial to set the temperature at 320 degrees f.

14. Press "start/pause" button to start.

15. When the unit beeps to show that it is preheated, open the lid.

16. Arrange the pan in "air fry basket" and insert in the oven.

17. Place the pan onto a wire rack to cool for about 10 minutes.

18. Carefully, invert the bread onto wire rack to cool completely before slicing.

19. Cut the bread into desired-sized slices and serve.

Nutrition: Calories 593 Total fat 32.6 g Saturated fat 14 g Cholesterol 59 mg Sodium 414 mg Total carbs 69.4 g Fiber 5 g Sugar 39.6 g Protein 11.2 g

Brown Sugar Banana Bread

Preparation time: 15 minutes

Cooking time: 30 minutes

Servings: 4

Ingredients:

- 1 egg
- 1 ripe banana, peeled and mashed
- ¼ cup milk
- 2 tablespoons canola oil
- 2 tablespoons brown sugar
- ¾ cup plain flour
- ½ teaspoon baking soda

Directions:

1. Line a very small baking pan with a greased parchment paper.
2. In a small bowl, add the egg and banana and beat well.
3. Add the milk, oil and sugar and beat until well combined.
4. Add the flour and baking soda and mix until just combined.
5. Place the mixture into prepared pan.
6. Press "power button" of air fry oven and turn the dial to select the "air crisp" mode.
7. Press the time button and again turn the dial to set the cooking time to 30 minutes.

8. Now push the temp button and rotate the dial to set the temperature at 320 degrees f.

9. Press "start/pause" button to start.

10. When the unit beeps to show that it is preheated, open the lid.

11. Arrange the pan in "air fry basket" and insert in the oven.

12. Place the pan onto a wire rack to cool for about 10 minutes.

13. Carefully, invert the bread onto wire rack to cool completely before slicing.

14. Cut the bread into desired-sized slices and serve.

Nutrition: Calories 214 Total fat 8.7 g Saturated fat 1.1 g Cholesterol 42 mg Sodium 183 mg Total carbs 29.9 g Fiber 1.4 g Sugar 8.8 g Protein 4.6 g

DEHYDRATED RECIPES

Cinnamon Apples Slices

Preparation time: 5 minutes

Cooking time: 12 hours

Servings: 4

Ingredients:

- 2 apples, core and sliced 1/4-inch thick
- 1/2 tsp vanilla
- 1/4 tsp ground nutmeg
- 1 tsp ground cinnamon
- 1/2 lemon juice

Directions:

1. Add apple slices, vanilla, nutmeg, cinnamon, and lemon juice into the zip-lock bag. Seal bag shakes well and let's sit for 10 minutes.
2. Arrange marinated apple slices on cooking pan in a single layer.
3. Place cooking pan in an omni toaster oven. Select dehydrate mode and set the omni to 135 f for 12 hours.
4. Serve and enjoy.

Nutrition: Calories 63 Fat 0.3 g Carbohydrates 16.1 g Sugar 11.8 g Protein 0.4 g Cholesterol 0 mg

Smoky Eggplant Bacon

Preparation time: 10 minutes

Cooking time: 4 hours

Servings: 4

Ingredients:

- 1 medium eggplant
- 1/4 tsp onion powder
- 1/4 tsp garlic powder
- 1 1/2 tsp smoked paprika

Directions:

1. Cut eggplant into the 1/4-inch thick slices.
2. Toss eggplant slices with onion powder, garlic powder, and paprika in a mixing bowl.
3. Arrange eggplant slices on cooking pan in a single layer.
4. Place cooking pan in an omni toaster oven. Select dehydrate mode and set the omni to 145 f for 4 hours.
5. Serve and enjoy.

Nutrition: Calories 32 Fat 0.3 g Carbohydrates 7.4 g Sugar 3.6 g Protein 1.3 g Cholesterol 0 mg

VEGETARIAN

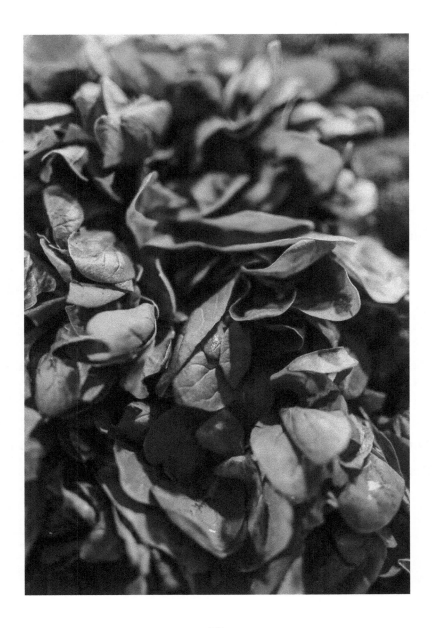

Beet, Tomato And Goat Cheese Mix

Preparation time: 30 minutes

Cooking time: 14 minutes

Servings: 8

Ingredients:

- 8 small beets, trimmed, peeled and halved
- 1 red onion, sliced
- 4 ounces goat cheese, crumbled
- 1 tablespoon balsamic vinegar
- Salt and black pepper to the taste
- 2 tablespoons sugar
- 1 pint mixed cherry tomatoes, halved
- 2 ounces pecans
- 2 tablespoons olive oil

Directions:

1. Put beets in your air fryer, spice them with salt and pepper, cook at 350 °f for 14 minutes and transfer to a salad bowl.
2. Add onion, cherry tomatoes and pecans and toss.
3. In another bowl, mix vinegar with sugar and oil, whisk well until sugar dissolves and add to salad.
4. Also add goat cheese, toss and serve.

Nutrition: Calories: 171 kcal/cal Total fat: 7 g Total carbs: 7 g Protein: 19 g Sugar: 4 g Fiber: 1 g Sodium: 582 mg Potassium: 259 mg

Broccoli Salad

Preparation time: 10 minutes

Cooking time: 8 minutes

Servings: 4

Ingredients:

- 1 broccoli head, florets separated
- 1 tablespoon peanut oil
- 6 garlic cloves, minced
- 1 tablespoon chinese rice wine vinegar
- Salt and black pepper to the taste

Directions:

1. In a bowl, mix broccoli with salt, pepper and half of the oil, toss, transfer to your air fryer and cook at 350 °f for 8 minutes, shaking the fryer halfway.
2. Transfer broccoli to a salad bowl, add the rest of the peanut oil, garlic and rice vinegar, toss really well and serve.

Nutrition: Calories: 171 kcal/cal Total fat: 7 g Total carbs: 7 g Protein: 19 g Sugar: 4 g Fiber: 1 g Sodium: 582 mg Potassium: 259 mg

Brussels Sprouts And Tomatoes Mix

Preparation time: 5 minutes

Cooking time: 10 minutes

Servings: 4

Ingredients:

- 1 pound brussels sprouts, trimmed
- Salt and black pepper to the taste
- 6 cherry tomatoes, halved
- ¼ cup green onions, diced
- 1 tablespoon olive oil

Directions:

1. Spice brussels sprouts with salt and pepper, put them in your airfryer and cook at 350 °f for 10 minutes.
2. Transfer them to a bowl, add salt, pepper, cherry tomatoes, green onions and olive oil, toss well and serve.

Nutrition: Calories: 171 kcal/cal Total fat: 7 g Total carbs: 7 g Protein: 19 g Sugar: 4 g Fiber: 1 g Sodium: 582 mg Potassium: 259 mg

Brussels Sprouts And Butter Sauce.

Preparation time: 4 minutes

Cooking time: 10 minutes

Servings: 4

Ingredients:

- 1 pound brussels sprouts, trimmed
- Salt and black pepper to the taste
- 1/2 cup bacon, cooked and diced
- 1 tablespoon mustard
- 1 tablespoon butter
- 2 tablespoons dill, finely diced

Directions:

1. Put brussels sprouts in your air fryer and cook them at 350 degrees
2. F for 10 minutes.
3. Heat up a pan with the butter over medium high heat, add bacon, mustard and dill and whisk well.
4. Divide brussels sprouts on plates, drizzle butter sauce all over and serve.

Nutrition: Calories: 171 kcal/cal Total fat: 7 g Total carbs: 7 g Protein: 19 g Sugar: 4 g Fiber: 1 g Sodium: 582 mg Potassium: 259 mg

Cheesy Brussels Sprouts

Preparation time: 10 minutes

Cooking time: 8 minutes

Servings: 4

Ingredients:

- 1 pound brussels sprouts, washed
- Juice of 1 lemon
- Salt and black pepper to the taste
- 2 tablespoons butter
- 3 tablespoons parmesan, grated

Directions:

1. Put brussels sprouts in your air fryer, cook them at 350 °ffor 8 minutes and transfer them to a bowl.
2. Heat up a pan with the butter over medium heat, add lemon juice, salt and pepper, whisk well and add to brussels sprouts.
3. Add parmesan, toss until parmesan melts and serve.

Nutrition: Calories: 171 kcal/cal Total fat: 7 g Total carbs: 7 g Protein: 19 g Sugar: 4 g Fiber: 1 g Sodium: 582 mg Potassium: 259 mg

SNACKS & APPETIZERS

French Fries

Preparation time: 10 minutes.

Cooking time: 16 minutes

Servings: 2

Ingredients:

- ½ lb. Potatoes, peeled and cut into ½-inch thick sticks lengthwise
- 1 tbsp. Olive oil
- Salt and ground black pepper, to taste

Directions:

1. In a large bowl, add all the listed ingredients: and toss to coat thoroughly.
2. Arrange the potato sticks onto a cooking tray.
3. Select air fry and then adjust the temperature to 400°f. Set the timer for 16 minutes and press start.
4. When cooking time is complete, remove the tray from the oven and serve warm.

Nutrition: Calories 138, fat 7.1 g, carbs 17.8 g, protein 1.9 g.

Air Fried Pickle

Preparation time: 10 minutes.

Cooking time: 18 minutes

Servings: 8

Ingredients:

- 16 dill pickle slices
- ¼ cup all-purpose flour
- Salt, to taste
- 2 small eggs, beaten lightly
- 1 tbsp. Dill pickle juice
- ¼ tsp. Garlic powder
- ¼ tsp. Cayenne pepper
- 1 cup panko bread crumbs
- 1 tbsp. Fresh dill, minced
- Cooking spray

Directions:

1. Place the pickle slices over paper towels for about 15 minutes or until all the liquid is absorbed.
2. In a bowl, mix the flour and salt.
3. In another shallow dish, add the eggs, pickle juice, garlic powder, and cayenne and beat until well combined.
4. In a third bowl, mix the panko and dill.

5. Coat the pickle slices with flour mixture, then dip into the egg mixture and finally coat with the panko mixture.

6. Spray the pickle slices with cooking spray. Arrange the pickle slices onto a cooking tray.

7. Select air fry and then adjust the temperature to 400°f.

8. Set the time to 18 minutes and press the start button.

9. Halfway, flip the pickles over and place them back into the oven.

10. When cooking time is complete, remove the tray from the oven and serve warm.

Nutrition: Calories 80, fat 2 g, carbs 6 g, protein 2.1 g.

Beef Taquitos

Preparation time: 10 minutes.

Cooking time: 8 minutes

Servings: 6

Ingredients:

- 6 corn tortillas
- 2 cups cooked beef, shredded
- ½ cup onion, chopped
- 1 cup pepper jack cheese, shredded
- Olive oil cooking spray

Directions:

1. Arrange the tortillas onto a smooth surface.
2. Place the shredded meat over one corner of each tortilla, followed by onion and cheese. Roll each tortilla to secure the filling and secure with toothpicks.
3. Spray each taquito with cooking spray evenly.
4. Arrange the taquitos onto a cooking tray.
5. Select air fry and then adjust the temperature to 400°f. Set the timer for 8 minutes and press start.
6. Turn the taquitos halfway.
7. When cooking time is complete, remove the tray from the oven and serve warm.

Nutrition: Calories 263, fat 10.7 g, carbs 12.3 g, protein 28.4 g.

Cheese Sandwich

Preparation time: 10 minutes.

Cooking time: 10 minutes

Servings: 2

Ingredients:

- 3 tbsp. Softened butter
- 4 white bread slices
- 2 cheddar cheese slices

Directions:

1. Spread the butter over each bread slice generously.
2. Place 2 bread slices onto a cooking tray, buttered side down.
3. Top each buttered bread slice with 1 cheese slice.
4. Cover with the remaining bread slices, buttered side up.
5. Arrange the sandwiches onto a cooking tray.
6. Select air fry and then adjust the temperature to 375°f. Set the timer for 10 minutes and press start.
7. Turn the sandwiches halfway.
8. When cooking time is complete, remove the tray from the oven.
9. Cut each sandwich in half vertically and serve warm.

Nutrition: Calories 307, fat 27.2 g, carbs 9.4 g, protein 8.2 g.

Perfect Cinnamon Toast

Preparation time: 10 minutes

Cooking time: 5 minutes

Servings: 6

Ingredients:

- 2 tsp. Pepper
- 1 ½ tsp. Vanilla extract
- 1 ½ tsp. Cinnamon
- ½ c. Sweetener of choice
- 1 c. Coconut oil
- 12 slices whole wheat bread

Directions:

1. Melt coconut oil and mix with sweetener until dissolved. Mix in remaining ingredients: minus bread till incorporated.
2. Spread mixture onto bread, covering all area.
3. Pour the coated pieces of bread into the oven rack/basket. Place the rack on the middle-shelf of the air fryer oven. Set temperature to 400°f, and set time to 5 minutes.
4. Remove and cut diagonally. Enjoy!

Nutrition: calories: 124; fat:2g; protein:0g; sugar:4g

DESSERTS

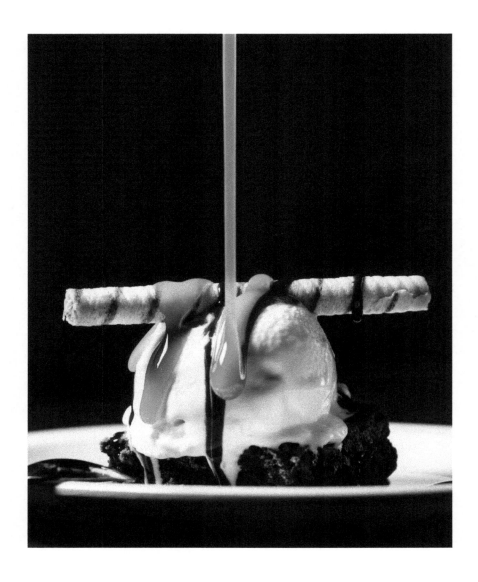

Vanilla Peanut Butter Cake

Preparation time: 10 minutes

Cooking time: 30 minutes

Servings: 8

Ingredients:

- 1 1/2 cups all-purpose flour
- 1/3 cup vegetable oil
- 1 tsp baking soda
- 1/2 cup peanut butter powder
- 1 tsp vanilla
- 1 tbsp apple cider vinegar
- 1 cup of water
- 1 cup of sugar
- 1/2 tsp salt

Directions:

1. Fit the cuisinart oven with the rack in position 1.
2. In a large mixing bowl, mix together flour, baking soda, peanut butter powder, sugar, and salt.
3. In a small bowl, whisk together oil, vanilla, vinegar, and water.
4. Pour oil mixture into the flour mixture and stir until well combined.

5. Pour batter into the greased cake pan.

6. Set to bake at 350 f for 35 minutes. After 5 minutes place the cake pan in the preheated oven.

7. Slice and serve.

Nutrition: Calories 264 Fat 1.8 g Carbohydrates 43.2 g Sugar 25.3 g Protein 2.6 g Cholesterol 0 mg

Moist Chocolate Brownies

Preparation time: 10 minutes

Cooking time: 20 minutes

Servings: 16

Ingredients:

- 1 1/3 cups all-purpose flour
- 1/2 tsp baking powder
- 1/3 cup cocoa powder
- 1 cup of sugar
- 1/2 tsp vanilla
- 1/2 cup vegetable oil
- 1/2 cup water
- 1/2 tsp salt

Directions:

1. Fit the cuisinart oven with the rack in position 1.
2. In a large mixing bowl, mix together flour, baking powder, cocoa powder, sugar, and salt.
3. In a small bowl, whisk together oil, water, and vanilla.
4. Pour oil mixture into the flour mixture and mix until well combined.
5. Pour batter into the greased baking dish.

6. Set to bake at 350 f for 25 minutes. After 5 minutes place the baking dish in the preheated oven.

7. Slice and serve.

Nutrition: Calories 150 Fat 7.1 g Carbohydrates 21.5 g Sugar 12.6 g Protein 1.4 g Cholesterol 0 mg

Yummy Scalloped Pineapple

Preparation time: 10 minutes

Cooking time: 35 minutes

Servings: 6

Ingredients:

- 3 eggs, lightly beaten
- 8 oz can crushed pineapple, un-drained
- 2 cups of sugar
- 4 cups of bread cubes
- 1/4 cup milk
- 1/2 cup butter, melted

Directions:

1. Fit the cuisinart oven with the rack in position 1.
2. In a mixing bowl, whisk eggs with milk, butter, crushed pineapple, and sugar.
3. Add bread cubes and stir well to coat.
4. Transfer mixture to the greased baking dish.
5. Set to bake at 350 f for 40 minutes. After 5 minutes place the baking dish in the preheated oven.
6. Serve and enjoy.

Nutrition: Calories 510 Fat 17 g Carbohydrates 85 g Sugar 71 g Protein 3.4 g Cholesterol 123 mg

Vanilla Lemon Cupcakes

Preparation time: 10 minutes

Cooking time: 15 minutes

Servings: 6

Ingredients:

- 1 egg
- 1/2 cup milk
- 2 tbsp canola oil
- 1/4 tsp baking soda
- 3/4 tsp baking powder
- 1 tsp lemon zest, grated
- 1/2 cup sugar
- 1 cup flour
- 1/2 tsp vanilla
- 1/2 tsp salt

Directions:

1. Fit the cuisinart oven with the rack in position 1.
2. Line 12-cups muffin tin with cupcake liners and set aside.
3. In a bowl, whisk egg, vanilla, milk, oil, and sugar until creamy.
4. Add remaining ingredients: and stir until just combined.
5. Pour batter into the prepared muffin tin.

6. Set to bake at 350 f for 20 minutes. After 5 minutes place muffin tin in the preheated oven.

7. Serve and enjoy.

Nutrition: Calories 200 Fat 6 g Carbohydrates 35 g Sugar 17 g Protein 3 g Cholesterol 30 mg

Lightning Source UK Ltd.
Milton Keynes UK
UKHW020630140621
385475UK00001B/15